THE MIRACULOUS VIRTUES OF VINEGAR

You knew vinegar was good for dressing up a salad and for making glass sparkle, but you're about to learn a whole lot more that you didn't know about this miraculous liquid.

You'll learn the celebrated 10,000–year history of vinegar and how it is made not only in America, but from fruits and grains by cultures scattered around the globe. You'll discover the many different varieties of vinegar, each with its own unique properties and personality, plus you'll be given step-by-step instructions on how *you* can brew a batch from scratch.

You'll find the preventive and curative benefits of vinegar through the trusted home remedies families have been using for generations to treat conditions from head to toe . . . from headaches to athlete's foot.

You'll learn that one splash of apple cider vinegar alone is an all-natural sour powerhouse containing key vitamins, over a dozen minerals, essential acids and several enzymes plus beta-carotene, nearly 30 nutrients and highly useful pectin.

Did you know you can even use vinegar as a cosmetic aid? After reading about how vinegar can help protect and beautify, you'll want to keep a bottle alongside your other beauty aids.

For cleaning and general maintenance, you'll learn the most popular formulas and money saving ways to use vinegar in every room in the house as well as outdoors.

The versatility of vinegar is deliciously demonstrated through cooking. So to leave you with a good taste in your mouth, Dr. Mindell has contributed a few of his favorite recipes, all of which call for vinegar as an ingredient.

Whenever and however you use vinegar—medicinally, for cleaning, or for cooking—after reading this Good Health Guide you'll most likely agree the virtues of vinegar are indeed miraculous. As miraculous and healthy as vinegar may be, however, it is only a part of a larger program of personal healthcare, which Dr. Mindell will share with you in a condensed form at the end of this Guide.

ABOUT THE AUTHOR

Earl L. Mindell, R.Ph., Ph.D. combines the expertise and working experience of a pharmacist with a researcher's grasp and a writer's skill in presenting facts about nutrition to an ever-widening audience for his books, articles, lectures and seminars. His *Vitamin Bible, Vitamin Bible for Your Kids, Food as Medicine, Herb Bible* and *Anti-Aging Bible* have been bestsellers.

Amazing Apple Cider Vinegar

The medicinal miracle, plus
the curative, cleaning and
cooking virtues of vinegars
from around the world

Earl L. Mindell, R.Ph., Ph.D.
with Larry M. Johns

KEATS PUBLISHING

LOS ANGELES

NTC/Contemporary Publishing Group

Amazing Apple Cider Vinegar is intended solely for informational and educational purposes and not as medical advice. Please consult a medical or health professional if you have questions about your health.

AMAZING APPLE CIDER VINEGAR

Published by Keats
A division of NTC/Contemporary Publishing Group, Inc.
4255 West Touhy Avenue, Lincolnwood (Chicago), Illinois 60646-1975, U.S.A.
Copyright © 1999 by Earl L. Mindell, R.Ph., Ph.D.
Printed and bound in the United States of America
International Standard Book Number: 0-87983-776-4
99 00 01 02 03 04 RCP 18 17 16 15 14 13 12 11 10 9 8 7 6 5 4 3

CONTENTS

THE HISTORY OF VINEGAR

Vinegar has been around in one form or another for at least 10,000 years. Through the ages it has served an important role as food preservative, condiment, cleaning agent, beauty aid and miraculous medicine.

The name vinegar is derived from the Latin word *vinum* meaning wine, and *acer* which denotes sharp or sour. Eventually the two words blended and became *vinegre*. In the Latin-root French language, the words "vin aigre" mean sour wine, and it is true that a wine left alone long enough can ferment and is said to have "turned to vinegar."

The Babylonians fermented the fruit of date palms, creating date vinegar, in 5,000 B.C. Vinegar residue has been scientifically traced to Egyptian urns in use as far back as 3,000 B.C. Vessels of vinegar figure prominently in early Greek and Roman artwork. Hippocrates, the father of medicine, prescribed vinegar for his patients.

The armies of Julius Caesar drank vinegar mixed with water as an invigorating tonic for its antiseptic benefits. Samurai warriors of Japan would down a vinegar-based beverage to accrue superior strength. The record of Hannibal's march over the Alps describes how vinegar was poured on hot boulders to crumble them to make way for his troops and elephants to proceed.

Eve had her encounter with an apple in the Garden of Eden, but did you know vinegar is mentioned no less than eight times in the Bible, four references in the Old Testament and four in the New Testament? Ruth 2:14 records, "And Boaz said unto her, 'At mealtime come thou hither, and eat of the bread, and dip the morsel in the vinegar.' " It is not certain whether Boaz was delivering culinary or medicinal advice.

During the time of Jesus Christ, vinegar was used as a condiment but was also valued for its medicinal properties. Jails in the holy land had two stone jugs kept near the wall where prisoners were flogged. One jug contained oil to soothe and heal, the other contained vinegar used as an antiseptic.

When it was mistakenly believed that it was acid in citrus fruit (rather than vitamin C) that cured scurvy, a ration of vinegar was issued to English sailors. During the American Civil War, soldiers with scurvy also received doses of vinegar.

IT'S IN THE AIR

Vinegar results when alcohol meets with air. More specifically, the oxygen in air interacts with tiny bacteria (vinegar bacillus) which also occur naturally in the air. The process, known as *acetous fermentation,* occurs in two stages. First, yeasts convert the sugar present in fruits and grains to alcohol. Then, bacteria convert the alcohol into acetic acid . . . this is what puts the "pucker" in vinegar.

It wasn't until 1864 that the famed French scientist, Louis Pasteur, discovered it was bacteria in vinegar that caused alcohol to turn into acid. Later, in 1878, a microbiologist (Hansen) actually isolated the three kinds of vinegar bacilli and accurately explained how they consume alcohol and excrete acid.

IT'S EVERYWHERE

Since ancient times, civilizations have allowed the bacteria which are in the air everywhere to turn whatever mildly alcoholic liquid was available into vinegars. While the overriding sour, puckery sensation of vinegar comes from the acid, fermentations result in different flavors and aromas ranging from the dark, sweet, expensive balsamic vinegars to the sharp, acid taste of the clear, cheap grain vinegars found in supermarkets. The potency of the pucker all depends upon the ingredients and the processes utilized.

In Europe it's no surprise to learn most vinegar is derived from grape wine. In China and Japan, vinegar starts with rice wine. In the Philippines, natives ferment coconuts. Vinegar in Mexico starts with cactus. Throughout Malaysia, it's pineapple that gets used. In the United States, most vinegar, and by far the most nutritious vinegar, is made beginning with apple cider. Other vinegar sources are molasses, sorghum, honey, maple syrup, melons, beets and potatoes.

AS AMERICAN AS APPLE VINEGAR?

Because apples are so universally available now, it's hard to believe they are not native to America. Actually it was the Pilgrims who first brought apple seeds with them from England in the 1600s. From then on early settlers all became Johnny Appleseeds, planting seeds and starting apple orchards of many types across the country. Today nearly 300 different varieties of apples grow in the 50 states and the fruit has become as American as apple pie.

Apple cider (from the French *sidre*) is the fermented juice of the apple. When apple cider, which is the first pressing of the apples, is heated to 170°F for ten minutes, you have apple juice. The heating, or pasteurization kills off the yeasts and bacteria which prompt fermentation. When you have *fresh* cider, it's a good idea to drink it within two weeks after opening the bottle because, once exposed to the air, it begins turning into vinegar.

HARD WINTERS, HARD CIDER

Early American settlers counted barrels of cider among their essential winter provisions, right up there with food and firewood. This wasn't apple juice. No, sir. This was hard cider, averaging about 6 percent alcoholic content. Perhaps the warming effects of fully fermented apple juice helped pass long winters in New England. It could explain why our colonial forebears started so many orchards. In other parts of the world today, cider is alcoholic and readily available, but in America hard cider is now hard to come by.

PLEASE PASS THE CIDER, TOM

In the early American colonies, consumption of cider was nothing short of prodigious. One Massachusetts settlement of only 40 families put up 3,000 barrels of cider for just one winter. About the same time in New Hampshire, an apple grower is reported to have brewed 4,000 barrels of cider, all of which was consumed in a nearby town prior to the next harvest.

Back then, cider was valuable currency in a prevailing barter economy. An 1805 diary records trading a half-barrel of cider for a child's schooling—liquid apples for the teacher I guess you could say.

The north orchard area of the Monticello estate of Thomas Jefferson was exclusively dedicated to advanced production of fine cider. Mr. Jefferson is said to have been particularly fond of the Virginia Hewes Crab and Golden Permian variety of apples for cider.

Hard cider, the kind with an alcoholic kick, was considered good for one's constitution and it is recorded that President John Adams would drink a glassful to start his day.

THE BIG BEVERAGE SWITCH

Up until the early 18th century, hard cider was the customary drink in America. The British had their beer, the French their wine but Americans had declared hard cider their natural beverage of choice.

By the early 19th century, however, the overwhelming popularity of hard cider with its 6 percent alcoholic content created two camps within the growing temperance movement. While some were out in orchards chopping down apple trees, others in the movement were serving cider at gatherings held to discuss the harmful consequences of Demon Rum, wild whiskey and those other nasty distilled spirits. Curiously, hard cider persevered through the Prohibition years and was one of the few exceptions to the Volstead Act. But by the time Prohibition was repealed, America somehow lost its taste for hard cider and began to substitute beer as its national beverage.

ABOUT VINEGAR

Vinegar is produced through the natural fermentation of almost any alcoholic liquid. In finished form, vinegar is mostly water with only two calories per tablespoon, zero fat and low sodium. Naturally fermented vinegars are a rich source of vitamins, trace elements and minerals including phosphorus, potassium, chloride, magnesium, sulfur, calcium and iron, along with healthful enzymes and acids. It is the *acetic* acid in vinegar which provides its characteristic puckering power or bite.

Vinegar possesses the same essential nutrients as the ingredients originally used to make it, but gains nutrients during the fermentation process, notably enzymes and amino acids. Many believe it is the natural fermentation process which endows the final product with its diverse healing properties. Later I will describe many of the remarkable if not miraculous medicinal applications attributed to apple cider vinegar.

When buying vinegar for health reasons, and for better taste, it is important to avoid the overprocessed, diluted, pasteurized, highly filtered, overheated brands. Study the label and search for pure, organic, aged (in wood not plastic), unfiltered, *less* attractive-looking varieties. You are more likely to find these better choices at health food and specialty stores than on supermarket shelves. And they will be higher priced. Plain distilled white vinegar will be the cheapest and the dark, aged-in-wood type will set you back as much as the best wines.

The apple cider vinegar you want will have the sharp aroma of apples, be full-flavored and have the robust color of the tannins from crushed cell walls of fresh, ripe apples. These naturally occurring preservatives in apples are what give cider vinegar its color as well as help contribute to its rich flavor. You're on the right track when your vinegar selection contains sediment on the bottom. Shake the bottle and if there is no sediment, some of the best part has been filtered out. If you cannot find the "good stuff," you may want to try making your own.

HOME SQUEEZIN'S

The easiest, most versatile and healthful vinegar to make at home is apple cider vinegar. You begin with fresh, whole apples from neighboring orchards, roadside stands or from a good food store. Use only pesticide-free varieties. If organic apples are not available, thoroughly wash the fruit to eliminate all traces of toxic chemicals and soil bacteria.

Apples that are green in color tend to taste tart and are generally crisp. Red apples are usually sweeter than green ones and may have a mealy texture. The sweeter the apples you use, the stronger the vinegar will be due to the higher sugar content. The more tart the apples, the sharper your vinegar will be. You'd like the cider mixture to have at least a 10 percent sugar content. Any single variety or mixture will do but if you can toss in a peck or two of crab apples, your cider will have just the right acidity and astringency.

For cider making, it's always best to pick, chop and press ripe, late-season apples, generally in October or around the time of the first frost in northern climates.

Like breaking eggs for omelets, to make vinegar you've got to crush a few apples. For this you'll need a sturdy apple cider press and a grinder. Just pour the clean, ripe, whole apples in the grinder. Apples are ground and emerge as a wet, golden brown mash, called "pomace." The ground-up apples are then squeezed and filtered through coarse cloth by slowly turning the screw on the press until rivulets of cider begin to flow. Collect the flow in gallon jugs.

At this point, if you didn't continue with your vinegar making, you'd have a lot of fresh squeezed apple cider. Mmm good! But don't stop now. You've collected good fresh organic apples, ground them up and pressed them. Now it really gets interesting.

All you do now is set aside the sweet cider, exposing it to air for six to eight weeks to do what comes naturally, which is to ferment to alcohol. You now have hard cider, which will then ferment *again* into the acetic acid solution we call vinegar.

What comes naturally, however, may not be all that palatable, due to the strains of bacteria out there. For this reason, the best way to insure good vinegar every time is to make hard cider, then rely on a "mother." A vinegar mother is the gummy mass of sour-smelling stuff floating on the top of a finished batch of vinegar.

"Mother of Vinegar" may be purchased at some health food stores, or you can start your own. Simply pour some hard cider into a pint-sized jar, cover with cheesecloth to keep out thirsty insects, and place in a warm dark place. At a temperature between 59 and 86°F, a sticky, stringy layer of mother will form and float on top in a few weeks. You'll know it's ready because it will give off the pungent smell of vinegar.

The cider should be placed in a wide-mouthed container (like a big wooden barrel) to expose a large surface of the hard cider to air. Cider matured in wood not only tastes better but will promote better fermentation.

Add the "mother" for faster conversion. Cover the container with several layers of cheesecloth or muslin to keep out dust and insects, but allow air through. When there is nothing left for the mother to live on (when all the alcohol has been converted to acetic acid), it will sink and die if not removed and saved to hurry along your next batch.

Vinegar should be made in a warm dark place. Expect the process to take several months. Aging will preserve the flavor found in a natural cider vinegar that is sadly sacrificed in the quick processing of most commercial brands. When the flavor seems right, strain off the vinegar and bottle it, sealing with a nonmetal stopper.

Acid test: The acid content of commercial vinegar is standardized at around 5 percent. However, you can expect an acid strength for homemade vinegar equal to the alcohol content of your hard cider. The percentage with homemade vinegar varies but if your hard cider was 6 percent alcohol it will convert to 6 percent acetic acid vinegar. If you really must know what the precise acidity of your vinegar is, you can use a wine-testing kit.

TYPES OF VINEGAR: EIGHT IS ENOUGH

The different types of vinegar present a fascinating array of colors, aromas, strengths, flavors and even textures that have, in some cases, been developed and refined over centuries from cultures and kitchens all over the world. There are eight types of vinegar:

1. White Vinegar
This is the clear, spirit vinegar that is not naturally fermented but distilled from common grains and is therefore referred to as "the vodka of vinegars." Other than its sharp acidic taste, this type of vinegar possesses no particular flavor of its own, which makes it useful for pickling cucumbers, beans or onions, and for use in strong sauces like salsa where added flavor is not necessary and even undesirable.

Because of its relatively high acid content of up to 13 percent and due to its low price, white vinegar is also commonly used for cleaning purposes.

2. Wine Vinegar

Vinegar, of course, is (or was) an adverse condition to wine-makers. But it wasn't long before enterprising wine-makers realized there might be a market for their bad luck. So in 1394, some French vintners established a guild of professional vinegar makers, the Corporatif des Maitres-Vinaigriers d'Orléans, in Orléans, France.

In the Orléans process, oak casks, three-quarters filled with wine, are laid on their sides, with small air holes on the top. Temperature is maintained at about 70°F. Vinegar mother forms on the surface, turning the alcohol into acetic acid which drops to the bottom of the cask. Wine vinegars made by this slow, natural process are expensive. Look at the label.

Good wine vinegar is clear, and if made from white wine, it is pale gold. When made from red wine, it is pink but lighter than the original wine. The taste is distinctly acidic, stronger than cider or malt vinegar, and the aroma will remind you of the wine from which it is derived.

3. Malt Vinegar

Malt vinegar has the same relationship to beer as wine vinegar has to wine. It is made from fermented malted barley. This type of vinegar actually has its origins in the northern European breweries as a way to get rid of bad beer.

Malt vinegar is particularly popular in England, where it is the traditional accompaniment to fish and chips. "Chips" are thick-cut fries. Sprinkling vinegar on them doesn't seem so strange when you realize ketchup is 10 percent vinegar.

Robust in taste, it contributes a hearty flavor and costs less than wine vinegars.

4. Rice Vinegar

The Chinese were making vinegar from rice wine 3,000 years ago. Rice vinegar can be red, black or white.

Naturally brewed rice vinegar is characterized by a light sweetness. It is full-bodied yet mild, providing a stimulating contrast of flavor that brings life to almost any food. A mainstay in salad dressings, pickling mixtures, and marinades it also perks up sauces, dips and spreads.

Traditionally brewed rice vinegars often contain a rice sediment, which, if disturbed, makes them look muddy. Rather than being a cause of concern, this sediment, as with other naturally produced vinegars, is a sign of quality.

5. Balsamic Vinegar

Balsamic vinegar, which comes from the province of Modena in Italy, has been made since the Middle Ages. Made from grapes with a high sugar content, the unfermented grape juice is boiled down to make a concentrated syrup which is cooled and transferred to a barrel, where it is then aged at least three years, but true balsamic vinegar is aged in aromatic woods for at least twelve years!

Balsamic vinegar is thicker than the usual vinegar, with a mahogany-like sheen. The exceptional flavor is mellow, deep and so sweet that the acid serves only to accentuate the herbal flavors picked up from the various aromatic woods in which the vinegar has been aged so long. The oldest balsamic vinegar—from 50 to more than 200 years old—are among the world's most expensive foods, on a price par with caviar and fine old cognac.

6. Sherry Vinegar

Sherry vinegar is made around Jerez in the southwest area of Spain which by no coincidence is also where great sherry is produced. The best sherry vinegars are aged for 20 to 30 years before bottling.

Usually available only in gourmet food or specialty stores, sherry vinegar is significantly higher priced than most wine vinegars yet far less expensive than bona fide balsamics. For this reason, many chefs regard sherry vinegar the best value among vinegars.

7. Apple Cider Vinegar

Apple cider vinegar is the most commonly used vinegar for home cooking. It is used primarily for adding "tang" as an ingredient in many delicious recipes from barbecue sauce to pie.

Of the eight different types of vinegar, apple cider vinegar is the one that reigns supreme for its medicinal and healing value. Because of this reputation, I will be discussing these properties in some detail in the next section.

8. Infused Vinegar
This type is any delicate or neutral-flavored vinegar steeped with herbs, garlic, berries and certain flowers.

MEDICINE CABINET MIRACLES

In medieval England, it was said, "To eat an apple before going to bed will make the doctor beg his bread." This evolved into the better-known saying, "An apple a day keeps the doctor away." And, as you'll learn in this section, the derivative of the apple—apple cider vinegar—would appear to keep not only the general practitioner away, but also the cardiologist, dermatologist, gastroenterologist, and even oncology doctors at bay as well.

Generations of families have used apple cider vinegar to help remedy such a wide variety of ailments, you could begin to believe vinegar is some kind of snake oil cure-all. Vinegar remains one of the most ancient and versatile medicinal mainstays the world has ever known.

On the following pages, I've noted some of the specific ailments both inside and outside the body which apple cider vinegar can prevent, diminish, alleviate or cure. I should emphasize that the focus here is on uses and applications of natural, unfiltered and preferably organic, *apple cider vinegar*. As with all things, even natural vinegar should be used in moderation.

Let's begin by highlighting some of the *internal* benefits that could derive from vinegar.

Have a Nice Daily Tonic

Who could argue that with a multitude of nutrients in every ounce, a little apple cider vinegar taken along with clean water would make an ideal tonic to start off each day? I certainly wouldn't. After all, it's just like taking a pure, natural multivitamin "pill" in liquid form that, at the very least, supplants deficiencies found in the processed, refined foods we encounter every day. A popular variation for a daily tonic is to add a teaspoon of honey to a glass of water containing one teaspoon of vinegar.

A summer "julep" of vinegar might prove particularly beneficial during the warmer months of the year when blood levels of lactic acid tend to increase.

Arthritis

Arthritis is one of the most common chronic diseases of aging found in Western countries. It is a condition of inflammation of the joints, which some researchers believe is caused in part by a buildup in the tissues of irritant metabolic wastes and toxins. People who are obese, who don't exercise much, who smoke, and who don't eat many vegetables, have a much higher risk of arthritis. Many arthritis problems can be solved simply by eliminating food allergies, the most common of which are wheat, dairy, corn and citrus foods.

Most natural treatments for arthritis involve a combination of diet, exercise and weight control. Nutrient-rich apple cider vinegar can play a dietary role in relieving the pain and in slowing the progression of arthritis. The prevailing remedy consists of one teaspoon of vinegar in a glass of water taken four times a day, sometimes with honey to make it a bit more palatable.

Asthma

According to some alternative medicine practitioners, asthma can be relieved by combining the nutritive values of apple cider vinegar with the benefits of accupressure by holding vinegar-soaked pads to the inside of wrists.

Them Bones

While it's not entirely clear how they work, it is acknowledged that trace elements needed to maintain bone mass and strength include manganese, magnesium and silicon, all of which occur in apple cider vinegar, and all of which are delivered to the body in a naturally balanced and easily-absorbable form. Doctors recommend supplements of these elements and others, particularly among post-menopausal women.

Cancer

To some degree cancer is a symptom of the harm created by free radicals—unattached, unwanted cells that wreak havoc wherever they lodge in the body. Antioxidants absorb free radicals, rendering them harmless. Beta-carotene, a carotenoid present in vinegar, is a powerful antioxidant. Moreover, carotenoids serve as the body's raw material for the production of vitamin A, another potent antioxidant, the scarcity of which has been linked, in particular, to cancers of the respiratory system, colon and bladder. Carotenoids and vitamin A work in concert to protect the body from cancers associated with chemical toxins.

The American Cancer Society recommends a high-fiber diet to help prevent several forms of cancer, particularly colon cancer. Pectin, a soluble fiber in vinegar, binds certain cancer-causing compounds in the colon, speeding their elimination from the body, according to a study published in the *Journal of the National Cancer Institute*.

Western Michigan University reports early test results which indicate vinegar can be used to increase the accuracy of conventional tests for cervical cancer. Adding the new vinegar-based test to the standard Pap test allows medical personnel to "... detect women at risk for cervical cancer who would not have been detected by the Pap test alone." The vinegar test is simple to administer, noninvasive, safe and low-cost.

Cholesterol

High blood cholesterol is a symptom and early warning sign of heart disease. The very best ways to lower cholesterol are by maintaining your ideal weight, getting plenty of exercise, eating plenty of vegetables and fruits, and avoiding processed foods, hydrogenated oils (found in margarine, baked goods, chips and many other processed foods) and other "nutrition-free" junk food.

One of the most effective ways of directly lowering cholesterol is to make sure there is plenty of fiber in your diet. Fiber is the indigestible portion of foods, and while all fiber is beneficial, not all fiber works the same way. Some fibers are water soluble and some are not. A water-soluble fiber soaks up water (adding bulk) and has the ability to interact with the body. Insoluble fiber also soaks up moisture but does not interact with the body. Fiber literally soaks up excess fats and cholesterol so that they are excreted from the body rather than reabsorbed.

In addition to fiber, in the form of pectin, vinegar also contains a number of amino acids which can neutralize harmful oxidized LDL cholesterol.

Colds

PH levels are a scale of acidity and alkalinity. It has been determined the pH levels of the body become more alkaline prior to the onset of a cold or flu. Since vinegar is acidic, taking a teaspoon in a half cup of water two or three times a day when a cold is coming on, can help rebalance pH levels, warding off the cold.

A folk remedy for a chest cold is to marinate a large square of brown paper (like a grocery store bag) in vinegar. Then, after it's soaked through, shake pepper on one side, bind it to the chest with strips of cloth (peppered side down on the skin). Remove after 20 minutes. At worst, the pepper might make you sneeze.

Constipation

Normal digestion includes the production of acid and pepsin by the stomach as well as digestive enzymes from the pancreas. As we age, we begin to underproduce these digestive juices, which can lead to constipation.

It is important not to ignore the problem because constipation interferes with the flow of nutrients throughout the body which keeps us healthier, longer. There are many diet and supplement therapies to address this problem, but the simplest and most effective is eating foods high in fiber to add bulk and stimulate proper bowel contractions. Fiber also stimulates the growth of healthful bacteria in the colon which aids in the assimilation of nutrients. As has been noted, apples and their fermented derivative, vinegar, contain the fiber pectin.

Coughs

Folk medicine holds that sprinkling the pillowcase with apple cider vinegar will soothe a dry night cough. Maybe you'd like to sleep on that.

Cramps

I've known many people who wake up during the night from the sharp pain of muscle cramps. The pains most often occur in the legs, but sometimes occur in the vicinity of the stomach or heart, which can be very scary!

When the cramps appear in the upper legs or feet, people will jump out of bed and start pounding the source of the cramp in an attempt to alleviate the pain. When the cramp is in the legs, many people are accustomed to getting up and "walking it out." Those plagued with nighttime leg cramps may find relief with a glass of water, fortified with one or two teaspoons of apple cider vinegar. Honey may also be added.

Diabetes

In the majority of individuals with diabetes, digestive impairment is present, which includes stomach malfunction with underproduction of hydrochloric acid and pepsin, as well as digestive enzymes by the pancreas.

When the stomach isn't performing as it should, the body cannot be well nourished with the protein and minerals it needs.

Cutting way back on refined sugars and carbohydrates, improving digestive function, plus vitamins and minerals, can make a big difference for diabetics. Physicians frequently recommend high-fiber diets to help control diabetes, and several studies have shown that pectin, the fiber in apple cider vinegar, helps control blood sugar (glucose) levels in diabetes.

Diarrhea

The pectin contained in apple cider vinegar provides effective antidiarrhea action because the fiber swells up to add bulk to the stool. In addition, intestinal bacteria transform pectin into a protective coating for the irritated lining.

Pectin is also effective against several types of bacteria capable of causing diarrhea. It's potent stuff. Pectin is the "pectate" in the popular over-the-counter diarrhea preparation, Kaopectate. It's so much less expensive and more natural to just take some apple cider vinegar!

Dietary Transition

People in the process of switching from a refined-food and/or meat-centered diet to one primarily composed of whole grains and vegetables, will benefit by taking a little vinegar to help the body manage the detoxification process and help it adjust to different digestion. During the early stages of transition, sip one-third cup of water mixed with one teaspoon of apple cider vinegar three times a day.

Depression

Eastern medicine believes that while mental depression is experienced in the mind, it is rooted in a stagnant liver. Due to its cleansing effect on the liver, mild cases of depression are thought to be relieved by taking a teaspoon of vinegar in a little water.

Others attribute the ability to decrease depression to its amino acid content.

Eyes

Vinegar's primary antioxidant—beta-carotene—contributes to maintaining good health by protecting the eyes from cataracts. Cataract development is related to oxidation of the eye's lens which occurs when free radicals alter its structure.

Fatigue

A buildup of lactic acid, released during exercise and stress, can cause fatigue, and the amino acids in vinegar can counteract the effect of excess lactic acid in the bloodstream. The enzymes and potassium in vinegar may also play a part in treating fatigue. One suggested dosage for chronic fatigue is three teaspoons of apple cider vinegar to an eighth of a cup of honey, taken at bedtime.

Food Poisoning

The antiseptic and disinfectant qualities of vinegar come into play in cases of nausea from eating overly fermented, old, or "bad" food. The vinegar neutralizes the poisons and kills harmful bacteria in the digestive tract. Take a quarter-teaspoon of apple cider vinegar once a day until food poisoning symptoms are relieved. Some doctors will recommend use of vinegar before meals when eating in foreign countries and visiting questionable restaurants.

Hiccups

If you *slowly* sip a glass of warm water with one teaspoon of vinegar mixed in it, hiccups will stop. This treatment works even better when you sip from the *far* side of the glass.

Gallstones and Kidney Stones

Vinegar is beneficial as a preventative and curative for kidney and gallstones. The theory is that the acids found in vinegar may serve to soften or dissolve the stones. One treatment, called a "gallbladder flush," involves eating only apples all day and then a cup of olive oil at bedtime. The following morning, stones are said to then pass in the stool. This ailment is said to be relatively unknown in areas or households where vinegar is frequently used.

Headache

A headache is a symptom and messenger telling you something is amiss in the body or mind that needs attention. The trouble may be in the liver, kidneys, gallbladder or other organs. It may be triggered by allergies and frequently by emotional stress. Vinegar is by no means a cure-all for all types of headaches, but it can be a very effective remedy for some.

Frequently when headaches strike, the urine, which is normally acidic, is more alkaline in nature. This indicates that the body is somewhat out of balance. Here the acids in apple cider vinegar may come to the rescue by helping the kidneys return to normal balance.

Inhaling vaporized apple cider vinegar may provide headache relief for some sufferers. In a pan from your kitchen, boil a splash or two of apple cider vinegar with some water. As steam begins to rise, remove from heat source and, with a towel over your head to act as a funnel, lean over the vapors and breathe in the steaming vinegar-water mixture. (Do not breathe in too deeply at first and burn yourself! Test the steam gently at first.) Alternatively, pour a dash of apple cider vinegar in an electric vaporizer and breathe the vapors for five minutes. With either method, expect results within half an hour.

Heart/Blood Pressure

The heart is a large muscle and works to pump blood through the arteries, vessels and tiny capillaries of the entire body. It's important to keep your blood pressure under control to prevent heart attacks and strokes. Dietary modifications (no salt, low-saturated fats, moderate coffee and alcohol) and taking apple cider vinegar with water several times a day, has been shown to lower blood pressure and strengthen the heart muscle. There is some evidence that vinegar acts as a blood thinner, reducing the risk of a stroke. The potassium in apple cider vinegar is also beneficial for the heart and blood.

Indigestion

Contrary to common belief, indigestion (and heartburn) are not due to *excess* stomach acid but, most often, a lack or *underproduction* of acid.

Normally our stomach digests food with strong hydrochloric acid and pepsin, an enzyme active only in an acid environment. When under-acidity is remedied by taking apple cider vinegar before a meal, the flow of nutrients to the body is improved, helping you feel more energetic and healthy.

Apple cider vinegar improves metabolism, due in part to the compatible presence of malic and tartaric acids which not only serve to restore the proper acid conditions, but also inhibit the growth of unfriendly bacteria in the digestive tract.

Apple cider vinegar has long been regarded a remedy for liver stagnation and accompanying indigestion. Vinegar appears to have highly activating and detoxifying properties. It counteracts the effects of rich, greasy food and functions as a solvent to break down fats and protein and dissolve minerals for improved assimilation.

For indigestion or to aid digestion, take one tablespoon vinegar in half a glass of warm water after, or preferably, before, a heavy meal. When taking *before* a meal, the vinegar solution acts to stimulate the flow of saliva which starts the digestion process in the mouth by activating digestive fluids to flow faster.

Muscle Soreness

Sore muscles and stiff joints may be the result of excess acid accumulation in the tissues and at body joints.

A dose of vinegar in water works in the body to precipitate the accumulated acid crystals, placing them in a solution which can then be flushed out of the body through the organs of elimination. The dosage called for is one to two teaspoons of apple cider in a glass of water. A spoonful or two of raw honey may be added.

Stiff joints may also be the result of a potassium deficiency. As noted earlier, you receive potassium when you take apple cider vinegar, helping to further relieve muscle soreness and aching joints.

To simply soothe tired or sprained muscles, sometimes just wrapping the afflicted area with a cloth wrung out of apple cider vinegar for up to five minutes will do the trick.

For all-over aching, soak in a tub of warm water into which you've poured two or three cups of apple cider vinegar. That's just *got* to make you feel better!

Nasal Congestion/Sinuses

Many suffer the discomfort of excess mucus from the nose or throat and from the sinus cavities. This annoying and painful drainage may be reduced for many by simply drinking one teaspoon of apple cider vinegar stirred in a glass of water. Lightening up on mucus-promoting foods (particularly dairy products) at the same time wouldn't hurt.

Nasal congestion can also be relieved by heating and inhaling a 50/50 mixture of vinegar and water.

Sore Throat

Causes of sore throat can be viral or bacterial. At the first sign of sore throat, send in germ fighting apple cider vinegar as a gargle consisting of a 50/50 solution of vinegar and warm water. For children you can add a little honey too if you need to, but do have them spit it out so they aren't unnecessarily swallowing germs. Gargle every hour or so until symptoms are relieved. Rinse the mouth (but *not* the throat) with fresh water to prevent any acid erosion of tooth enamel.

If you are susceptible to sore throats (or want to avoid laryngitis), it's a good idea to gargle the apple cider vinegar solution once or twice a week to ward off germs in the throat.

Ulcers

A controlled test study, published in the *Japanese Journal of Pharmacology*, indicates vinegar as mild as 1 percent concentration may prompt the gastric system to mount a natural defensive action to protect the stomach from alcohol-induced damage. Additional research proving vinegar can prevent stomach ulcers caused by alcohol has yet to be conducted. However, since this early study appeared to offer over 95 percent protection from these types of ulcers, the possibility that vinegar may someday be used as an ulcer preventative looks promising.

Yeast Infection (Candida)

Yeast infections, also called candida, can be local, usually in the vaginal area, or more widespread. When strictly local, the infection can be controlled or eliminated with a variety of local applications.

Yeast normally exists in harmony with other organisms in the body, but when something alters the usual pH of the vagina, it can cause the yeast there to grow at a high rate, causing itching and burning sensations. Many things can disturb the balance of yeast, most notably, antibiotics and diet.

As a very effective preventative and curative, you can use a vinegar-and-water douche. Changing the pH of the vaginal environment at the first sign of a yeast infection may be sufficient to end the condition. Standard procedure is to douche twice a day with a solution of two tablespoons of vinegar to one quart of room temperature water until symptoms disappear.

OUTSIDE THE BODY

You've heard the "inside" story on vinegar, now let's turn our attention to its external values.

Bleeding

Vinegar stops bleeding by helping the blood congeal. For nosebleeds, soak a cotton ball in apple cider vinegar and stuff gently up the nostril(s). Tilt the head back slightly and pinch the nose while breathing through the mouth, for up to five minutes. Then slowly remove the cotton. Repeat the procedure as necessary.

Burns

Straight, undiluted apple cider vinegar, right from the bottle, will lessen the pain and soreness of burns, including sunburns, when applied to a burn on the skin.

Cuts and Abrasions

Cuts and abrasions are less likely to become infected when swabbed with vinegar. Healing is faster among people who use vinegar with regularity.

Ears

"Swimmer's ear" is a condition accompanied by itching, pain and even temporary hearing loss. It can be caused not only by swimming but by showering. You can seek relief from "swimmer's ear" and the possibility of developing ear infections, by dropping three or four drops of vinegar, diluted with water or alcohol in equal parts, in the ear after swimming or if you notice water blocking your ears after a shower.

Feet

To control foot odor, soak feet a couple of times a week in one-third cup of vinegar added to a small pan of warm water.

When bothered by the peeling and itching of athlete's foot, soak feet in 50/50 solution of vinegar and water for about ten minutes a day up to ten days or until symptoms disappear. Resume treatment as necessary.

Hair and Scalp

One of the causes of an itching scalp and dandruff are bacteria which clog hair follicles, forming dry crusts. The acid and enzymes present in apple cider vinegar kill the offending bacteria. Some people believe it is a fungus which causes dandruff, but vinegar will kill those too! Pour full-strength vinegar on the head and wrap with a towel for an hour before washing hair. Repeat this procedure as necessary.

For an after-shampoo rinse that will leave the hair shiny, less frizzy and with more body, mix one part vinegar to four parts water.

Vinegar can be used very effectively to treat ringworm of the scalp. Ringworm is a fungus which is transmitted directly from child to child but may also be transmitted to children from cats and dogs. Massage apple cider vinegar with the fingertips into the ringworm area on the scalp three times a day, beginning each morning and continuing through to bedtime.

Herpes

To relieve the pain and discomfort of both cold sores and genital sores, apply apple cider vinegar, direct from the bottle, to the affected areas of the skin where the sores are located. The itching and burning discomfort will rapidly dissipate after the vinegar is applied, and the sores will heal more quickly.

Insect Bites and Stings

If you're going on a picnic or to the beach, pack your sunscreen *and* apple cider vinegar. Apple cider vinegar has long been used to stop the itching and pain caused by many-legged biters and stingers like mosquitoes and bees. Vinegar also inactivates the venom of stinging jellyfish. Repeatedly apply full strength directly on the affected area or use a compress.

Poison Ivy and Poison Oak

A mixture of equal parts of apple cider vinegar and water or rubbing alcohol relieves the itching caused by poison ivy, poison oak or nettle stings. Just dab it on the affected area.

Shingles (Herpes Zoster)

To relieve the pain and discomfort of shingles, apply apple cider vinegar, direct from the bottle, to the affected areas of the skin where the shingles are located. The itching and burning discomfort will rapidly dissipate after the vinegar is applied, and the shingles will heal more quickly.

Sunburn

Although it is important to get some direct exposure to the sun so that your body can produce vitamin D, sunburn is something you should avoid to prevent skin cancer later in life. Avoiding sunburn will also mean less wrinkled skin as you age, and fewer "age spots." To relieve sunburn pain, sponge the skin gently with apple cider vinegar. Leave it on to prevent blistering and peeling.

Weight Control

Folk medicine has it that a single teaspoon of apple cider vinegar in a glass of warm water before each meal will melt away excess pounds.

No one knows for sure how this regimen works, but it may be because a) it really does burn calories; b) it takes the edge off the appetite; or c) just fills the stomach. No matter. The effect is the same: less food over the lips means less on the hips (or wherever the pounds tend to go on your body).

Apple cider vinegar is also beneficial for underweight conditions due to its ability to help the body digest, assimilate and use food better.

BODY BEAUTIFUL

We've covered the internal and external medicinal virtues of vinegar but the miracle doesn't cease there. Vinegar also possesses cosmetic properties to make you look better from head to toe and, as a result, make you feel better too.

The condition of your skin can mirror the health of your body. The skin is your largest organ, weighing an average of about 15 percent of your total body weight, and covering an area of six square feet. Skin protects your underlying tissues from harm; helps to control body temperature; responds to environmental stimuli; sweats out water, salts, and toxic compounds; and synthesizes vitamin D. The skin requires a constant supply of many nutrients because it is composed of rapidly dividing cells which are sensitive to nutrient status. Two reasons why vinegar is so good for skin is that it's nutrient rich and has a pH which is nearly the same as healthy skin.

Varicose Veins

The unsightliness of varicose veins can be overcome by wrapping the legs with cloth dampened with apple cider vinegar. With the legs elevated, leave the cloth on for half an hour in the morning and at night. Shrinking of the veins can be expected within six weeks. To accelerate results, follow each application with a glass of warm water with one or two teaspoons of apple cider vinegar in it. Drink slowly.

Facial

To prevent and eliminate facial blemishes and acne, steam clean your face by using a towel trap over your head and placing your face over a steaming pan of vinegar water. One-quarter cup of vinegar to the quart. Once pores are open, gently wipe apple cider vinegar over the face with a cotton pad to loosen dirt and oil. Repeat steaming but conclude process by splashing face with 50-50 solution of cool vinegar and water to close pores. Steam clean weekly or more often as needed.

Rubbing the skin gently with a coarse towel after first steaming will help remove old, dry scales that have loosened and will leave your skin looking fresh and youthful.

Corns and Calluses

Soak feet in a shallow pan of warm water with a half cup of apple cider vinegar, for half an hour. Rub down corns and calluses with a clean pumice stone.

Nails

I prefer that you don't use nail polish, because it is made from very toxic materials which can be absorbed through the skin. But, if you do, nail polish will stay on longer and go on smoother when fingernails are first cleaned with white vinegar before applying the polish.

Hair

To brighten dark hair and highlight blond hair, use a vinegar-and-water rinse. (Earlier I mentioned how a vinegar rinse will control dandruff and leave hair shiny and healthier.) A final vinegar rinse after shampooing will also eliminate the frizz for those sporting a new permanent, and will prevent buildup of hair control additives (sprays and gels).

CUPBOARD COMPANIONS

As versatile and miraculous as vinegar is all by itself, there are times when its healing powers are enhanced by combining it with companions from the cupboard. Vinegar's most faithful companion is honey. A few of these cupboard couplings are listed here.

Bee Aware of Honey!

Honey is food collected and predigested by bees. The nectar from thousands of flowers is processed into a thick, luscious liquid composed mostly of simple sugars dextrose (pure glucose) and levulose. In addition, honey is packed with amino acids, trace elements, enzymes, protein, phosphorus, carbohydrates, calcium, niacin, potassium and iron. It's a golden, saturated, liquid multivitamin pill. And honey requires no refrigeration since it is naturally antiseptic and will not support the growth of mold or bacteria.

Sour vinegar and sweet honey. Who says opposites don't attract!

Sore Throat
Mix one-fourth cup honey with one-fourth cup apple cider vinegar and take one tablespoon every four hours for the relief of sore throat pain.

Sipping a syrup of one-half cup each of apple cider vinegar and water, three tablespoons of honey and one teaspoon of cayenne pepper, will speed healing and ease the discomfort of a sore throat.

Upset Stomach
Calm an unsettled stomach by sipping a glass of warm water mixed with one tablespoon of honey and one of apple cider vinegar. This solution will also minimize gas.

Cough
Halt nagging, hacking coughs by taking a mixture of one-half cup honey and a tablespoon of vinegar. My grandmother used to also add a dash of brandy or whiskey.

Blood Pressure
A dose of two tablespoons of vinegar and two tablespoons of honey in a glass of water with breakfast each day is believed to normalize blood pressure while lowering cholesterol.

Arthritis
The favored vinegar tonic for dealing with arthritis is one teaspoon honey and one teaspoon apple cider vinegar, mixed into a glass of water and taken morning and evening. Expect results within a month.

Skin

Oily skin can be helped with a regular facial mask made with brewer's yeast and enough liquid (use water or skim milk) to form a paste. Apply to freshly cleaned skin, rinsed with vinegar water. Pat on and allow to completely dry before rinsing off with warm and then cool water. Blot face dry.

Itchy skin and hives can be eased by applying a paste of cornstarch and vinegar. Just pat on. The itching is drawn out as the paste dries.

Fade age spots (liver spots) by wiping them every day with blend of two teaspoons of vinegar and one teaspoon onion juice. Apply on spots with cloth or sponge. In a few weeks, the spots will begin to fade.

Protect skin from harsh summer sun or windburn by applying a protective coat of apple cider vinegar and olive oil mixed half and half. Helps prevent sunburn and chapping.

Condition skin while you sleep by mixing one-fourth cup apple cider vinegar with three large mashed strawberries and let sit for two hours. Strain off the flavored vinegar and apply the juice to face and neck. The following morning, wash off. Skin will be more radiant and soft.

Deep clean skin with ingredients from all over the kitchen. Take: 1 egg yolk; 1 teaspoon apple cider vinegar; 1 teaspoon lemon juice; ¼ cup olive oil; 1 teaspoon baking soda. Thoroughly mix egg, vinegar, lemon and oil. Add the baking soda and stir. Apply and massage well on skin with fingertips. Rinse with warm water and pat dry.

Hair

Regularly have a glass of water containing two teaspoons of apple cider vinegar, and one teaspoon each of honey and molasses, for a full head of richly nourished hair.

MIRACLES AROUND HOME SWEET HOME

Many commercial household cleaning products are harmful to the environment and to your wallet. Take a stroll with me through the house while toting an ordinary spray bottle of white vinegar and I'll show you safe, nontoxic ways to clean, deodorize and disinfect—dirt cheap.

For cleaning purposes, put away the good stuff and use inexpensive clear vinegar. It will cut grease, soap scum, inhibit mold, dissolve mineral buildup and retard bacteria growth wherever used. If you have any concerns about the effect of vinegar on surfaces, test out a small area first. If the smell bothers you, just add a squeeze of lemon.

Ready to really clean up? Good. Let's stand in the family room.

IN THE FAMILY ROOM

Perhaps the most well-known cleaning use of vinegar is for making windows sparkle. Use full-strength white vinegar and spray on windows. Dry right away with a soft, clean cloth. For light maintenance, you can use a diluted formula of one-fourth cup vinegar to a quart of water.

For uncarpeted floors clean enough to eat off, add a cup of vinegar to a bucket of water. Or, after using another floor cleaner, rinse floors with this vinegar-water solution to get up all residue that could dull the finish.

Light carpet stains can be removed by rubbing a paste of two tablespoons of salt and one-half cup vinegar into the stain and allowing it to dry before vacuuming. For tougher stains, add two tablespoons of borax to the paste before rubbing it into the carpet.

Pet accidents happen, and when they do, pour undiluted vinegar directly on the stain and wipe clean with strong strokes. Blot with cold water. The area is cleaned and sufficiently deodorized so the pet will not return to the scene of the crime.

Furniture or woodwork that may have grown cloudy over the years can be brightened by rubbing with a solution of one tablespoon of clear vinegar in a quart of warm water. Buff to a luster using a soft dry cloth.

If coaster-challenged guests have left white rings from wet glasses on furniture, they'll go away (the rings, not the guests) when you rub them with a mixture of equal parts white vinegar and olive oil.

Iodine works to heal scratches on wood too. Just a little iodine one-to-one with vinegar is all it takes. Apply with small artists' watercolor paint brush. More iodine deepens color and more vinegar will lighten color.

Wipe down Dad's vinyl easy chair or any other vinyl surface with a combination of one-half cup each vinegar and water and two tablespoons of liquid soap. Rinse off with fresh water and buff dry.

Those toys lying around can be easily disinfected with a wee bit of vinegar and some hot water with a little soap. Rinse toys well after cleaning.

Leave the room smelling fresh by adding one teaspoon baking soda to one tablespoon of vinegar in two cups of water. After the foaming action subsides, pour into a spray bottle, shake well and spritz it into the air for a fresh fragrance. (Simmering a pot of water with about one-fourth cup vinegar will also sweeten air.)

IN THE LAUNDRY ROOM

Stepping into the laundry room and on over to the washing machine, add one full quart of vinegar and run for a complete cycle. This will dissolve accumulated soap scum from the tub and drain hoses for cleaner, trouble-free washing.

It's a good idea when washing clothes for the first time, to add a cup or two of white vinegar during the rinse cycle to help remove original manufacturing chemicals and their accompanying smell.

For routine washing, add one-fourth cup clear vinegar along with detergent for brighter colors and whites. The vinegar also serves as a fabric softener and will inhibit germ growth, including athlete's foot germs on socks. (If you suspect bright colors may run, immerse the garment in full-strength white vinegar to set color before washing. Test a spot first.)

A rinse with vinegar added will end static cling and even cut down the lint clothes sometimes pick up during washing.

Perspiration odor and stains in clothes will disappear when presoaked overnight in three gallons of water mixed with one-fourth cup vinegar.

Stains on washable fabrics caused by grass, wine, berries, cola, coffee or tea may be removed if full-strength vinegar can be applied to the spot within 24 hours and then washed as usual.

Ink stains on clothes can be removed by soaking in milk for one hour, then covering with a paste of vinegar and cornstarch. When the paste dries, wash clothes as usual.

If there is any body odor emanating from that shirt or blouse you wanted to wear, sprinkle the armpits with vinegar and iron it. Fresh as a daisy!

And look at that iron. Any starch buildup making it stick? Wipe the sole plate when cold with full-strength white vinegar. Then to keep an iron free of mineral deposits, once in a while fill the water reservoir with straight white vinegar and steam iron clean with an old towel or rag. Repeat using water. Rinse out iron thoroughly.

Light scorch marks on clothes may be removed by gently rubbing them with undiluted white vinegar, then wiping with a clean, white cloth.

Hem marks left after altering hemlines or letting out

seams may be gently rubbed with a cloth dampened in white vinegar, then steam ironed. No telltale lines!

IN THE BATHROOM

Ducking into the bathroom, sponge chrome and stainless steel fixtures with straight vinegar, then buff to a shine with a damp soft cloth.

Wipe down ceramic or plastic surfaces with vinegar diluted with an equal amount of water. (Avoid using vinegar on marble because it may erode it.)

For the toilet bowl, pour in a cup of undiluted white vinegar. Let it stand for about five to ten minutes then flush away the unsightly ring. For a tougher toilet cleaner, first pour vinegar on a stain then shake a little borax over the vinegar. Give it two hours to soak. Brush then flush. The results will bowl you over.

Tackle tub and tile soap film with straight vinegar, wiping surfaces, then rinsing with water. For water scale buildup, mix one-fourth cup vinegar with one teaspoon alum. Wipe the mixture on surfaces and scrub with a small brush. Don't forget to brush the solution into a showerhead to dissolve clogged minerals. Rinse with water and buff dry.

It's easy to keep plastic shower curtains free of ugly mold and mildew. Just put them through a short rinse cycle with a cup or two of vinegar. Do not put through dryer. For maintenance, spray the curtains between washings with a 50/50 mix of vinegar and water.

To clean combs and hairbrushes, soak them for fifteen minutes in two cups hot soapy water mixed with one-half cup vinegar. Rinse clean in fresh water.

IN THE KITCHEN

That bottle of vinegar you have stored in the kitchen is there for cleaning, too. Countertops and appliances will shine streak-free just by wiping them with a soft cloth well-dampened with straight white vinegar. For extra gleam, dry surfaces with a paper towel.

For extra-greasy places, mix one-fourth cup vinegar with two cups hot water and stir in a teaspoon of borax. Pour the mixture in a spray bottle, spritz it on then wipe with dry cloth. This is a good solution to use on exhaust fan grills.

Freshen the microwave by bringing a cup of water with one-fourth cup vinegar in it to a boil on your microwave oven's highest setting. Set the temperature setting to "low" and boil for three minutes. Dry all interior surfaces and door. This leaves your microwave sparkling clean and deodorized.

Perk up the taste of your coffee by dissolving the lime and mineral deposits that are caked onto the heating elements of your electric coffee maker. Every so often, fill the reservoir with white vinegar and run through the brew cycle. Twice if necessary. Rinse with two cycles of plain water. Your coffee maker is ready to brew faster, better tasting coffee.

Remember how clean vinegar gets your windows? The same goes for your glassware. Just half a cup of vinegar in the dishwashing water helps eliminate water spotting. You can also put a cup of vinegar on the bottom rack of your automatic dishwasher for spotless results.

Stainless steel pots and pans come up bright when scrubbed with a little paste of baking soda and vinegar.

When you're stuck with stuck-on food, soak or simmer the cookware for a few minutes in two cups water and one-half cup vinegar. This will soften the harder food and speed cleanup.

If you're using a sponge for kitchen cleanups, you can renew it by soaking overnight in a quart of hot water mixed with one-fourth cup vinegar. The next day, the sponge will be clean, deodorized and germ-free.

It's a good idea to wipe down wood cutting boards at least once a week with full-strength white vinegar. You can also sprinkle and rub the wood with baking soda, then spray with vinegar, letting sit for five minutes. The bubbling action cleans, deodorizes, and disinfects the boards. Rinse off in clear water.

Kitchen drains will remain odor-free and free-flowing by pouring a handful of baking soda down the drain followed by a half cup of white vinegar. Cover for ten minutes, then run water down the drain. Whenever odor alone is the problem, just pour a half cup in the drain.

For the garbage disposal, grind through a tray of undiluted vinegar ice cubes. Flush with cold water. Your disposal is now clean and fresh.

Smelly fish and fresh cut onions are nothing to cry about when you simmer a little vinegar in water in an uncovered pot. The offensive smell will be absorbed. Stale or smoky odors will also be absorbed by an open bowl of vinegar sitting out in the kitchen.

IN THE GARAGE

Here we are in the garage and there's the car. Spritz all the chrome parts on the car with vinegar and watch that chrome shine.

And, hey, look on the windshield . . . a decal that expired three years ago. Soak it off with vinegar. Dissolves that chewing gum on the floormat as well.

Remember when you have to leave your car out in the freezing temperatures, coat the windows with a mixture of three parts vinegar to one part water to keep windows frostfree.

Look at those hardened paint brushes over there. The old dried paint can be softened by covering the bristles with boiling vinegar and letting them stand for an hour. Keep in mind when painting: vinegar absorbs paint odors.

Projects that require removing rusty blots or mineral accumulation can be cleaned up by soaking or applying full strength vinegar to the affected area. One-fourth cup of vinegar in a quart of water will clean metal screens, storm doors and aluminum lawn furniture.

See those leather work shoes in the corner caked with salt? Clean them up by wiping them off with a cloth drenched with vinegar, then buffing with a dry cloth. To preserve the leather, mix together one tablespoon each of vinegar and alcohol, one teaspoon of vegetable oil or beeswax, and one-half teaspoon liquid soap. Heat ingredients and when cool, work the mixture over the surface. Then brush until shoes are radiant with new life.

IN THE GREAT OUTDOORS

If you'll walk outside with me I can show you even more cleaning-with-vinegar tricks.

First, before you put on your sunglasses, remember to clean them with vinegar water just as you do windows.

Stepping outside, you may see weeds and grass growing in the driveway and in cracks where you don't want them to grow. Pour on a little vinegar for a safe alternative to toxic chemical products.

When working with garden lime, splash your hands with undiluted vinegar to neutralize the rough drying effects. Follow the dousing with a rinse of water from the hose.

When you cut flowers and take them inside and put them in a container, first add two tablespoons of white vinegar to a quart of warm water. When stems are immersed in this solution, the flowers will last much longer.

If you spot ants where you don't want them to be, spray a mixture of equal parts vinegar and water at possible points of entry—windowsills, door jambs, thresholds and at any foundation breaks. Ants will avoid the area and you will have avoided using pesticides.

Don't forget as mentioned earlier, that you can stop the pain and itching of insect bites and nettle stings you might get outside by applying straight apple cider vinegar directly on the affected area.

MIRACLES ON THE MENU

Have you ever noticed how complementary cranberry sauce is with turkey? Or apple sauce with roast pork? Or a slice of lemon with fish? A mushroom with steak? People naturally crave these accompaniments because they contain natural acids which help break down fats and protein, tenderize the meat and cause gastric juices and saliva to flow, which aids in digestion. (Mushrooms are rich in citric acid, in case you were wondering.)

The acidic content of vinegar isn't the only good reason Americans consume millions of gallons of vinegar every year. Vinegar's acids tenderize vegetables like cabbage, beets, carrots and broccoli; prevent enzymatic browning (foods that darken when exposed to air produce an off flavor); kill and inhibit growth of bacteria (especially important with foods not intended for immediate consumption, e.g. deviled eggs or potato salad on picnics); and make beans and other legumes more digestible and less gas producing.

Vinegar serves to balance the effects of salts you ingest and also dulls the craving for sweets. Vinegar itself contains only two calories per tablespoon and is free of fat and sodium.

In most kitchens, vinegar is an indispensable ingredient with endless culinary uses. To demonstrate the versatility of vinegar, the recipes that follow span the menu, starting with a vinegar cocktail and ending with my personal favorite pie, all containing that miraculous ingredient.

To begin, let's all have a *Rosy Red Vinegar Cocktail*:

ROSY RED VINEGAR COCKTAIL

1 quart tomato juice, chilled
1½ tablespoons red wine
  vinegar
1 white onion, grated
2 tablespoons honey

1 teaspoon garlic salt
2 tablespoons basil leaves,
  chopped
Freshly grated black pepper

Combine all of the above in a large pitcher and mix thoroughly. Chill for at least one hour, allowing flavors to intermingle. Pour into short, frosty cold glasses, garnished with a wedge of lemon on the rim. Serves 6.

Ahhh . . . refreshing cocktail, huh? Nonalcoholic and good for you. Whets the appetite for an appetizer of *Sweet 'n' Sour Meatballs*.

SWEET 'n' SOUR MEATBALLS

1 small can pineapple, crushed
  (8 oz.)
½ cup apple cider vinegar
¼ cup brown sugar, firmly
  packed
2 tablespoons soy sauce
½ teaspoon freshly grated
  ginger
1 ½ pounds ground beef, lean
  (or 1 pound beef and ½
  pound sausage)

¾ cup cracker crumbs
¼ cup milk
1 egg, slightly beaten
1 teaspoon salt
Dash freshly grated black
  pepper
1 tablespoon olive oil
1 tablespoon cornstarch
1 tablespoon water

Drain can of pineapple and set aside, saving juice. Add enough water to saved juice to make ¾ cup. Add vinegar, soy sauce and ginger; set aside.

Mix meat with crumbs, milk, egg, salt and pepper. Form small meatballs using rounded tablespoons for each. In a large frying pan, brown meatballs in oil. Add pineapple liquid, cover and simmer for 15 minutes or until meatballs are done, stirring every five minutes. Stir in pineapple. Combine cornstarch and water and then pour into pan. Heat until sauce thickens, occasionally stirring. Enough for 6.

For the soup course, let's agree to have a healthy *Cold Gold Soup*.

COLD GOLD SOUP

3 large peaches, ripe
½ cup orange juice, fresh
  squeezed
2 teaspoons honey
2 drops Tabasco sauce

White pepper
1 tablespoon balsamic vinegar
1 tablespoon mint, finely
  chopped
orange peel

Peel peaches and cut into small chunks. Add honey and orange juice. Blend until smooth. Stir in Tabasco and white pepper, cover and chill at least one hour.

Stir in vinegar and chopped mint, then ladle soup into chilled bowls. Garnish with fresh whole mint leaves and zests of orange peel. Serves 3.

For our salad, a fresh bunch of mixed bitter greens with the dressing would be nice and healthy.

HONOLULU LULU DRESSING

6 tablespoons red wine vinegar
3 tablespoons water
2 tablespoons fresh lemon juice
2 tablespoons pineapple juice
¼ cup honey
½ teaspoon dry mustard

6 drops Tabasco sauce
¼ teaspoon celery seed
1 garlic clove, finely chopped
⅓ cup olive oil
black pepper freshly ground

Stir together the first four liquid ingredients. Add honey, mustard, Tabasco, celery seed and garlic. Whisk in the oil and fresh pepper. Cover and chill overnight for maximum "lulu" flavor. Yields about one cup.

For an entree, may I suggest a *Poached Chicken and Pasta Salad with a Basil Vinaigrette Dressing?*

POACHED CHICKEN AND PASTA SALAD
WITH BASIL VINAIGRETTE DRESSING

Basil Vinaigrette

2 egg yolks, room temperature
2 tablespoons Dijon mustard
1⅔ cup extra virgin olive oil
½ cup basil leaves, chopped

¼ cup apple cider vinegar
Black pepper, freshly ground
⅓ cup water, warm

Blend egg yolks and mustard in food processor. With beaters turning, very slowly add olive oil. Process until mixture emulsifies then blend in the vinegar. Add pepper, basil and water.

Poached Chicken

2 whole chicken breasts,
    boneless and skinless
Cold water
1 tablespoon white wine

Salt and pepper
1 bay leaf
Fresh sprigs of parsley and
    thyme

Combine water, wine, salt, pepper, bay leaf and sprigs of parsley and thyme in large pot. Add chicken breasts, bring to simmer and cook until breasts are tender. Remove from heat and allow to cool in liquid. When cool, cut breasts into thick strips.

Salad

1 pound salad-style pasta,
    cooked
1 cup snow peas
1 cup green beans
1 red bell pepper

1 cup cherry tomatoes
⅓ cup basil, diced
1 teaspoon thyme leaves
Salt and black pepper

Steam peas and beans until slightly crunchy. Cut open pepper, remove seeds and membranes and slice into strips. Halve the tomatoes.

Assembly: Dump pasta into large bowl, add chicken strips, bell pepper, tomatoes, basil, thyme, salt and pepper. Pour dressing over top and toss lightly. Permit to sit one hour. Before serving, mix in snow peas and beans. Garnish with fresh basil. Serves 6.

VINEGAR PIE

When offered on the menu, this dessert is one that is the second most popular variety ordered by patrons of the restaurant where I obtained this recipe. Apple is the favorite but this *Vinegar Pie* is my personal favorite:

1 pie shell, baked
1 cup butter, softened
1 cup sugar
2½ tablespoons apple cider
   vinegar

6 eggs
2 teaspoons vanilla

Cream together butter and sugar. Add in vinegar, eggs and vanilla. Beat well and pour into pie shell. Bake at 350 for about one hour or when top is golden brown all over.

FRUIT VINEGAR CORDIAL

For after dinner, a cordial of *Fruit Vinegar* provides the finishing touch.

Rinse one cup pitted cherries then place them in a jar. Add one tablespoon sugar. Pour a pint of warm red wine or apple cider vinegar over the cherries, seal the jar and allow to stand about two weeks before straining and bottling. Makes one pint.

MAXIMIZING YOUR HEALTH: MY COMPREHENSIVE PLAN

Forget about calendar years. Growing older is not in itself detrimental. Many symptoms associated with advanced years are simply the end result of a lifetime of neglect accompanied by natural nutritional deficiencies which can be forestalled if not remedied.

The body is self-healing and self-correcting when you give

it a chance. Many degenerative diseases are affected by what you decide to eat and drink and how you choose to live. While it's true heredity creates certain tendencies, *you are still in control of maximizing your health.* You can start feeling better in just days by making the right choices.

I'm pushing sixty and I'm not on high blood pressure medicine, heart drugs, or prostate medication. My weight is about where it should be, and my energy level is terrific.

Over the past 25 years I've developed a simple yet comprehensive plan anyone can gradually adopt at any time when they decide to maximize their health. Regardless of age or current condition, my plan will strengthen your overall health, prevent illness and prolong your life.

The basic elements of my plan are as follows:

Eat Whole Foods

When you eat processed and refined foods, your body will shout, "I am what you eat." Your body doesn't need, nor does it know how to handle, commercially packaged foods which are devoid of natural nutrients but full of additives, dyes, sugar, salt, artificial sweeteners and hydrogenated oils.

Switch to whole foods; foods just as they come from gardens, orchards and the sea. When you eat a variety of fresh vegetables, fruits, grains, beans, fish, meat, and poultry, you're getting healthy doses of the vitamins and minerals and other natural nutrients you need to combat symptoms of aging.

Drink Good Water

Water is an overlooked essential nutrient. By "good," I mean pure plain H_2O. Designer waters, coffee, tea and soft drinks are not water substitutes. Good, clean water isn't from the tap either, because that's as processed as some packaged foods. Get yourself a good home filtration system and drink six to ten glasses a day.

Eat More of the *Right* Food

You've heard it before but I recommend that you cut down on your consumption of meat and dairy products which contain too much saturated fat. Low-fat protein alternatives are fish, turkey and soy products. Also eat more complex carbohydrates, which contain protein plus fiber. Some choices are vegetables, grains and beans.

Cut way back on sugar! It's disguised in a lot of foods and the crimes it commits, or is an accessory to, include most chronic diseases, including heart disease, diabetes and arthritis.

Reduce or Avoid Reliance on Drugs

I'm talking about *all* kinds of drugs—prescription, over-the-counter, so called "recreational"—all incur side effects that can threaten your health and even your life.

Get A Move On

Movement is exercise. Let me stress there is absolutely no need for you to embrace strenuous, heavy sweating to achieve the benefits of exercise. Just move. Make any physical activity you do a "workout," from housework to yard work. Don't avoid any activity that involves moving your body. Try to fit in a brisk walk of 30 minutes *at least* five days a week. Your stress level will decrease, your energy will increase.

Adopt A Supplemental Health Plan

The kind of "insurance" I'm talking about here you don't get from a broker or agent but from vitamins and minerals. You simply cannot get all your body requires strictly from the foods you eat, either because they are insufficient in quantity or because the foods are missing in your menu altogether.

Not everyone requires the same vitamins and minerals, but here is my basic program, which you can then adapt. There are many multiple vitamins available that will give you the dosages listed below. Look for one that dissolves easily, is small enough to swallow easily, that uses natural not synthetic vitamins, and that doesn't use starch or colorings.

Ideally, you'll take a high-potency multiple vitamin at least twice a day that gives you:

Vitamins
- Beta-carotene or carotenoids, 10,000–15,000 IU
- The B vitamins, including:
  (thiamine), 25–50 mg
  (niacin), 25–100 mg
  (riboflavin), 25–100 mg
  (pantothenic acid), 25–100 mg
  (pyridoxine), 50–100 mg
  B-12, 500–1,000 mcg
  biotin, 100–300 mcg
  choline, 25–100 mg
  folic acid, 200–400 mcg
  inositol, 100–300 mg
- Vitamin D, 100–500 IU
- Vitamin C, 500–3000 mg
- Vitamin E, at least 400 IU total per day

Minerals
- Boron, 1–5 mg
- Calcium (citrate, lactate or gluconate), 100–500 mg (women should take a total of 600–1,200 mg daily)
- Chromium (picolinate), 200–400 mcg
- Copper, 1–5 mg
- Magnesium (citrate or gluconate), 300–500 mg (women should take a total of 300–600 mg daily)
- Manganese (citrate or chelate), 10 mg
- Selenium, 25–50 mcg
- Vanadium (vanadyl sulfate) (25–200 mcg)
- Zinc, 10–15 mg

Since vitamin C, vitamin E, calcium and magnesium tend to make a multivitamin larger, you can take a multivitamin with smaller amounts of those vitamins and then take the others separately. A calcium/magnesium combination works well at bedtime when it will help you relax and prevent leg cramps.